PLANTEIN

A VEGAN ATHLETE´S GUIDE - HOW TO COMBINE PLANT BASED FOODS TO REACH OPTIMUM PROTEIN NUTRITION

By

SCOTT OTERI

Table of Contents

Introduction

More and more people are becoming vegetarians and vegans. It is not without a reason. Food coming from animal sources is scientifically proven to be bad for us. So why do we still eat it. It is because of ignorance. We were not so familiar that plant food sources are as protein rich as the animal sources, but way better for our health. It is particularly hard for athletes. They have a larger need for protein intake than normal people. So in this book we will get you familiar with everything you need to know about proteins and amino acids. But our focus will be on your health. After a long research, everything you need to know about plant based food is in one place.

You will have no problem beating the meat with this book and you will be healthier than ever. If you are an athlete, you will find out what is the best way to boost your performance and which plant food to combine to have enough protein for all of your needs. Highlight of this book is the table with food combinations for 100% bioavailability. You don't have to pay for expensive nutritionist to make your diet regime or waste your time with some suspicious advices. With this book you can do it all by yourself, and of course, meat free.

The meat based food is a thing of past. A lot of people have figured that out, and it is time for you to do the same. So lean back, and enjoy in this guide.

All the basics about Protein

To get started, I would like to get you familiar with some technicalities. The first thing is the proteins.

From the chemical point of view, proteins are large biological molecules, or macromolecules, consisting of one or more long chains of amino acid residues. Proteins perform a vast array of important functions within living organisms, including catalyzing metabolic reactions, replicating DNA, responding to stimuli, and transporting molecules from one location to another. Proteins differ from one another primarily in their sequence of amino acids, dictated by the nucleotide sequence of their genes, and which usually results in folding of the protein into a specific three-dimensional structure that determines its activity.

We said there are a lot of functions of proteins. Aside from water, proteins are the most abundant kind of molecules in the body. The most important ones are that protein is the building material for our muscles, skin, bones and a lot of other tissues in the body. If there is some damage to any of our tissues, protein is necessary in rebuilding that same tissue. Protein is also crucial for building new tissue, a characteristic very important to children in their development and to pregnant women. So for you as an athlete it is up most important to track your protein intake. Only in that way you will be able to achieve the goal you are streaming towards.

They are also regulators of balance in our bodies for fluid and acid, and that keeps us safe from a lot of life threatening situations like swelling or drying up. Also one more important function is clotting of blood, preventing our blood to drain out when we cut ourselves.

On top of that, proteins are among the components of enzymes, antibodies, and hormones. They all have a big role in many processes in the body that, like digesting your food or fight disease. Proteins also carry important nutrients through our body. One example is hemoglobin, blood protein that carries oxygen from our lungs to our cells. And in the end, without another source, body can convert protein to energy.

The time of day in which you provide your body with protein is also important. So here is the best time to do it:

- First things first, before the workout. That allows you to build more muscle. It needs some time for the proteins you have taken to start working, so it is best to do it before the workout. In that way they have the time to settle.
- Have your protein intake after a workout. That is because your muscles need nutrition so they could recover and grow.

- Before sleeping. Person sleeps 5 to 8 hours per day on average. That's a long time without protein. And although you are sleeping, your body is still functioning on a high pace.
- After you wake up. Body has consumed the protein during sleep and you need to refill that.

Also there is a lot of debate out there about combining your carbs and protein intake. The fact is that your body works better when there is a balance of carbs and protein. It is more healthier to combine protein and carbs than to separate them. "The pairing of protein and carbs is what fills you up the most and gives you the energy. The combination of carbs and protein right after a workout helps you to replace stored carbs that are consumed by workout. The best food for you, nuts, seeds, legumes consists of protein and carbs. So, strive to balance your protein and carbohydrate intake.

Protein in food

Functional properties of proteins in food are related to their structural and other physicochemical characteristics. A fundamental understanding of the physical, chemical and functional properties and the changes these properties undergo during processing is essential if the performance of protein in food is to be improved and if underutilized proteins, such as plant proteins proteins, are to be increasingly used.

Protein plays important role in the expression of sensory attributes of foods. Food preferences by costumers are predominantly based upon color, flavor, texture of the food. Protein is one of the major ingredient that contributes to these properties. For example, the textural properties of bakery products are manifestation of the viscoelastic properties and dough forming properties of wheat gluten. Muscle proteins impart unique textural characteristics to meat.

Regarding the protein in food, most food contains some protein. What people mostly don't know is that the plant food is an awesome source of protein, so if you are vegan that will be great for you. Some of them are the legumes, grains, some vegetables, nuts and seeds. Legumes, or called pulses in certain parts of the world, have higher concentrations of amino acids and are more complete sources of protein than whole grains and cereals. Examples of plant foods with protein concentrations greater than 7 percent include soybeans, lentils, kidney beans, white beans, mung beans, chickpeas, cowpeas, lima beans, pigeon peas, lupines, wing beans, almonds, Brazil nuts, cashews, pecans, walnuts, cotton seeds, pumpkin seeds, sesame seeds, and sunflower seeds.

There are plenty of reasons to eat more meat-free meals: They're nearly always cheaper, lower in calories, and better for the environment. It's easy to get enough protein without eating animals, but the doubters often have another concern: Are these meat-free protein sources complete? Well they are, and there is no reason not to use them. Meat is doing more bad things to you than good, so if you have a choice, always strive towards plant proteins.

There are also manufactured protein sources called protein powder. Protein powders – such as casein, whey, egg, rice and soy – are among them. These protein powders may provide an additional source of protein for bodybuilders. The type of protein is important in terms of its influence on protein metabolic response and possibly on the muscle's exercise performance. The different physical and/or chemical properties within the various types of protein may affect the rate of protein digestion. As a result, the amino acid availability and the accumulation of tissue protein is altered because of the various protein metabolic responses.

A major portion of the world protein supply comes from plant proteins. Although plant proteins are cheap and abundant, direct consumption of these proteins in conventional foods is very limited, mainly because of lack of desirable functional behavior. It is estimated that about 8 kg of plant proteins is needed to produce one kg of animal proteins.

How much Protein do you really need ?

Most people don't know what their daily protein intake should be. Pilling up proteins isn't always a good thing. Consuming too much of it, will result in taking more calories and fat than the body needs. Also high intake of protein can lead to increased water loss due to common urination. Normal person should aim to get between 10 and 35% of their daily calories from protein.

Of course there are some categories that need more. So the rules about how much protein can body absorb doesn't apply for everyone in the same way. It's all about the individual. Protein needs increase in people who are physically active, as well as in elderly ones and people who are recovering from injuries. That brings us to athletes. They need significantly more proteins, and here is why.

For best results, a diet high in protein is beneficial for muscle growth. Most sports involve physically breaking down and tearing muscle during the activity and repairing it afterward. Because of that, protein needs of active people are mandated by the length, frequency, and intensity of their workouts. Athlete's needs for protein intake depend on various factors. First there is a type of athlete, body weight, does he tends to loss or gain weight, intensity and duration of exercise and the age.

Endurance athletes such as marathon runners need about 50% more protein than a normal person, according to sports dietitian Josephine Conolly-Schoonen.

If you are wondering how much protein do endurance athletes exactly need to consume, here it is. It was believed that 75 grams 70 kg person per day was enough. However, studies have shown that figure should be about 100–112 grams. That means around 1,5 is needed.

To find out how much you require, multiply your weight in kilograms by 1.4 to 1.7, depending on your exercise intensity. This gives you the amount of protein that you should consume on a daily basis.

Body Builders need twice as much protein as a normal person. The greater the number of hours in training and the higher the intensity, the more protein you need.

But like everything, protein intake has its limits. It isn't without importance if you take too much protein. It can cause some serious side effects.

Eating more protein than your body needs can interfere with your health and fitness goals in a number of ways, including weight gain, extra body fat, stress on your kidneys, dehydration, and leaching of important bone minerals.

If you eat more protein than your body requires, it will simply convert most of those calories to sugar and then fat. Increased blood sugar levels can also feed pathogenic bacteria and yeast, such as Candida albicans (candidiasis), as well as fueling cancer cell growth. Excessive protein can have a stimulating effect on an important biochemical pathway called the mammalian target of rapamycin (mTOR). This pathway has an important and significant role in many cancers. When you reduce protein to just what your body needs, mTOR remains inhibited, which helps minimize your chances of cancer growth.

Additionally, when you consume too much protein, your body must remove more nitrogen waste products from your blood, which stresses your kidneys. Chronic dehydration can result, as was found in a study involving endurance athletes.

There are a few studies that have shown that too much protein can do you more harm than good. The first study was led by Valter Longo, a professor at the University of Southern California, who counts longevity and cell biology among his areas of expertise.

He and his colleagues showed that high protein consumption is linked to increased risk of cancer, diabetes and death in middle-aged adults, although this was not the case for older adults who may benefit from moderate protein consumption. Also, the effect is much reduced when the protein comes from plant sources.

The second study was led by Stephen Simpson, a professor at the University of Sydney in Australia, whose group works at the interface of physiology, ecology, and behavior. From studying mice, he and his fellow authors concluded that diets low in protein and high in carbohydrates are linked to the longest lifespans.

Both studies suggest it is not just calories, but also diet composition - particularly in terms of amount and type of protein - that may determine the length and health of a lifespan.

Prof. Longo says:

"We studied simple organisms, mice and humans, and provide convincing evidence that a high-protein diet - particularly if the proteins are derived from animals - is nearly as bad as smoking for your health."

High-protein diet had highest risk, except in older adults.

In their study, Prof. Longo and colleagues analyzed data on over 6,800 American adults who took part in the National Health and Nutrition Examination Survey (NHANES) III, a US national survey that assesses health and diet.

They found that:

The researchers found that consuming a high-protein diet in middle age significantly increases the likelihood of dying from cancer or diabetes.

Participants aged 50 and over who said they ate a high-protein diet were four times more likely to die from cancer or diabetes, and twice as likely to die from any cause, in the following 18 years.

Those who consumed moderate amounts of protein had a three-fold higher chance of dying of cancer.

These effects either reduced or disappeared altogether among participants whose high-protein diet was mainly plant-based. However, in those aged 65 and over, the effect was nearly the opposite - high protein intake was linked to a 60% reduced risk of dying from cancer and a 28% reduced risk of dying from any cause, with similar effects for moderate protein intake.

The researchers defined a high-protein diet as one where at least 20% of the calories consumed come from protein. Cell experiments have suggested the amino acids that proteins are made of can reduce cellular protection and increase damage to DNA, both of which might explain why high-protein intake is linked to cancer.

Complete and incomplete proteins

Complete proteins contain a balanced set of essential amino acids for the human organism. Except the meat and dairy products (which bring some unwanted side effects), plants such as soybeans, quinoa, buckwheat, hempseed, and amaranth are great source of complete proteins.. The net protein utilization is seriously affected by the limiting amino acid content (the essential amino acid found in the smallest quantity in the food stuff), and also affected by the salvage of essential amino acids in the body.

Incomplete proteins are low or lacking one or more of the amino acids we need to build cells. Combining various incomplete proteins, you can get a complete one.

Amino Acids

Surely you have heard a thousand times the expression: Aminos or Amino Acid. But did you ever thought what is behind that expression. When proteins are digested or broken down, amino acids are left. Amino acids are organic compounds that combine to form proteins. The precise amino acid content, and the sequence of those amino acids, of a specific protein, is determined by the sequence of the bases in the gene that encodes that protein. The chemical properties of the amino acids of proteins determine the biological activity of the protein.

Amino acids have an influence on the function of organs, glands, tendons and arteries. A large scale of our cells, muscles and tissue is made up of amino acids, meaning they carry out some of the most important body functions, like determining cells structure. Beside playing a key role in the transport and the storage of nutrient, also they are furthermore essential for healing wounds and repairing tissue, especially in the muscles, bones, skin and hair as well as for the removal of all kinds of waste deposits produced in connection with the metabolism.

Many doctors have now confirmed that a supply of amino acids (also by way of nutritional supplements) can have positive effects. The importance of amino acids for human well-being is on the increase. By providing the body with optimal nutrition, amino acids help to replace what is lost and, in doing so, promote well-being and vitality.

The amino-acid pool is solely responsible for achieving a balanced metabolism. The amino acid pool is considered to be the entire amount of available free amino acids in the human body. The size of the pool deviated, but it is believed to be around 120 to 130 grams in an adult male. If we consume protein in the diet, the protein in the gastro-intestinal tract is broken down into the individual amino acids and then put back together again as new protein. This process is called protein biosynthesis. Our whole amino acid pool is transformed, or changed three to four times a day, meaning that the body has to be supplied with more amino acids, partly by protein biosynthesis, partly by the diet or through consumption of suitable dietary supplements.

The objective is that the amino acid pool is complete and maintained in the correct combination. If the one or more amino acids are not available in sufficient quantities, the production of protein is smaller and the metabolism will only function in a limited way. And for an athlete, that is never a good thing.

As a negative consequences of a limited supply of nutrients you can experience weight problems, hair loss, skin problems, sleep disorders, mood swings and/or erectile disorders but also arthritis, diabetes, cardiovascular imbalance (high cholesterol levels, high blood pressure) or even menopausal complaints.

There are many of them:

Amino acids are classified into three groups:

Essential amino acids

Nonessential amino acids

Conditional amino acids

Essential amino acids – the ones you must obtain

Humans can produce 10 of the 20 amino acids. Failure to obtain enough of even 1 of the 10 essential amino acids, those that we cannot make, results in degradation of the body's proteins—muscle and so forth—to obtain the one amino acid that is needed. Unlike fat and starch, the human body does not store excess amino acids for later use—the amino acids must be in the food every day. Essential amino acids can't be made by the body. . Plants, of course, must be able to make all the amino acids. Humans, on the other hand, do not have all the the enzymes required for the biosynthesis of all of the amino acids. As a result, we must get them from the food we eat.

The essential amino acids are histidine, isoleucine, leucine, lysine, methionine, phenylalanine, threonine, tryptophan, and valine. These amino acids are required in the diet.

Histidine promotes growth and the repairing of body tissues.

Isoleucine is necessary for protein synthesis, and is found in all foods that contain complete protein (especially in plants). In one study it proved that deficiency of Isoleucine has produced loss of muscular coordination in lab rats, as well as a hypersensitivity to pain, heat, and cold.

Leucine is found in some plants and other high protein foods. It is needed for protein synthesis, and a good functioning immune system.

Lysine found in legumes. It is necessary for protein synthesis, and is integral to the production of Carnitine, which in turn is essential to the oxidation of fatty acids in the body. Lysine is the limiting amino acid in wheat.

Methionine have a primary function is to facilitate fat and protein metabolism; the body also uses it to manufacture Cysteine, another amino acid. Methionine is found in legumes and other vegetables.

Phenylalanine is used by the body use to produce tyrosine, a nonessential amino acid, and three important hormones (Epinephrine, Norepinephrine and Thyroxine) as well as melanin (brown skin pigment). Phenylalanine uses the same active transport channel as tryptophan to cross the blood-brain barrier; and, in large quantities, it interferes with the production of the brain neurotransmitter, Serotonin.

Threonine plays a major role in the synthesis of purines, which in turn break down uric acid, a by-product of protein digestion. Threonine is also necessary to bodily processes requiring Glycine, a non essential amino acid.

Tryptophan is a precursor of Niacin (Vitamin B3), and of Serotonin, the brain neurotransmitter that regulates appetite, pain, mood, and sleep. Because of Tryptophan's mood-elevating, sleep-inducing capabilities, it is prescribed as both a sleeping agent and an antidepressant.

Valine is essential in the growth and maintenance of body tissues (found in fibrous animal proteins).

Semi-essential Amino Acids

Cysteine, although once considered a non-essential amino acid, has been re-classified as semi-essential. This is because if there is a deficiency of Methionine (an essential amino acid) in the diet, the body can use Cysteine in place of Methionine to synthesize protein. Good sources of Cysteine include fowl, soybeans, oats, and wheat. Food manufacturers use Cysteine as an antioxidant to protect the Vitamin C content of processed foods. Also, bakers mix Cysteine into dough to speed kneading. Cystine, on the other hand, is used as a dough strengthener as well as a dietary supplement and works as a detoxifier in the body, but also performs as an antioxidant, combating free-radicals. It also strengthens stomach lining and is essential to healthy hair, skin and nails.

Tyrosine was also originally classified as a non essential amino acid, but is now considered semi-essential by most nutritionists, because if the body gets a sufficient amount, it can be used in place of phenylalanine to synthesize protein. Legumes are good sources of tyrosine. The brain uses tyrosine to manufacture Norepinephrine, an "upper" that boosts mental alertness.

Non–essential amino acids – your own body makes them

Non-essential amino acids are those that can be synthesized by the body and are different from essential amino acids that are obtained from food. The term 'non-essential' does not infer that those amino acids are any less important however. The body is simply capable of creating them on its own; therefore it is not necessary for it to attain them from an outside source. These nonessential amino acids serve many functions to create optimal health.

Alanine

During exercise, muscle tissue breaks down and toxins are released. Alanine works to remove these toxins so the liver is able to metabolize them and eliminate them from the body. Alanine may also help to keep cholesterol levels in check.

Asparagine

A requirement in amino acid transformation, asparagine helps the nervous system maintain its equilibrium. It also acts as a detoxifier in the system and regulates metabolism.

Aspartic Acid

Similar to asparagine, aspartic acid helps to elevate metabolic levels. Due to its effect on cellular energy, it is sometimes used to combat fatigue and depression. Aspartic acid also acts as a synthesizer for other amino acids.

Cystine

Created from the formation of two cysteine molecules, and therefore regarded as a more stable amino acid, cystine also works as a powerful antioxidant and helps to form strong connective tissues. Cystine is one of the amino acids responsible for the creation of glutathione, a vital liver detoxifier, and has been used in topical treatments to maintain youthful-looking skin.

Glutamine

Also aiding in the production of glutathione, glutamine is the most abundant amino acid in the bloodstream. Proper brain function and digestion require glutamine as does the immune system. Studies have also shown glutamine may possibly help to suppress hunger.

Glutathione

Made up of cystine, glutamine and glycine, glutathione is an amino acid that is found within all cells and affects virtually every system in the body. It has anti-aging properties, improves brain function and protects cells from oxidative stress. Glutathione may also lower blood pressure, improve sperm count in males and help in the treatment of certain types of cancer.

Glycine

A glucogenic amino acid, glycine supplies beneficial glucose the body needs for energy. It is essential for proper cell growth and function, and is also crucial to digestive health. Glycine makes up a large portion of collagen which helps skin retain its elasticity and healing properties.

Histidine

Important in the production of red and white blood cells, histidine helps to repair body tissue. Histamine is produced by histidine during an allergic reaction, and also is responsible for sexual arousal. Like many other amino acids, histidine is also a detoxifier.

Proline

In order for the body to create new, healthy cells, it produces proline. This amino acid helps in the regeneration of skin and helps to reduce sagging and wrinkles. Also a proponent of collagen and cartilage, proline helps keep muscles and joints pliable.

Serine

Also derived from glycine, serine is essential to brain function, particularly the chemicals that determine mood and mental stability. Serine, found in all cell membranes, also aids in muscle formation and immune health.

Taurine

Like glutamine, Taurine is a free amino acid that travels through the bloodstream and is also a detoxifier and digestion aid. It has also been shown to improve brain function and athletic performance.

Threonine

A protein balancer in the body, threonine helps to form tooth enamel, stabilize blood sugar levels and assists in healthy liver function. It also acts as a stress reducer and skin rebuilder.

Sources of Non-Essential Amino Acids

Although these nonessential amino acids are readily available in a healthy human body, they can also be found in whole foods like nuts, grains, meats, fruits and vegetables, or can be added to the body through supplements should there be a deficiency. Careful monitoring of supplements is advised to avoid altering the normal balance of citric acid in the system causing the liver and kidneys to function improperly.

Amino Supplements – The real deal

Supplements can do wonders for you regardless of what you are using them for. For athletes, supplements can be part of the training solution, allowing them to train harder, recover faster, and decrease down time due to overtraining and injuries. But to accomplish these things, it is important to take the right supplements at the right time and in the right amounts.

Amino acid supplements can offer health and fitness benefits. Supplements that include all the amino acids found in whole-food proteins can serve as a substitute for this macronutrient. Choosing to consume some of your protein in this manner can help ensure your diet does not lack any specific amino acid. These supplements can be especially beneficial during times of illness or when you are recovering from an injury and your overall protein needs are elevated. Amino acid supplements are be helpful if you eat only plant-based proteins, which may lack one or more essential amino acid - but that should not be a problem as you normally combine different sources of plant based protein.

The advantage of taking amino acids as supplement is that amino acids have been already broken down and can be absorbed more easily into the bloodstream. Food needs to be broken down and digested before the amino acids from the protein can be assimilated. It is possible that you will not use all of the protein you consume from food sources. So amino supplements can increase your protein intake. An effective way to take amino acid supplements is to include them with every meal.

One of the best and easiest ways to get amino supplement is by drinking protein drinks. They contain high quality protein that you need to recover and build muscle. Providing you with essential amino acids right after your workout will do magic for your muscles. Some of these drinks have additional ingredients, like minerals and vitamins that can increase uptake and delivery of amino acids to the muscle cells. Others provide added glutamine or branched-chain aminos.

In addition to amino acid supplements that contain all 20 amino acids, there are also supplements for branched-chain aminos. The branched-chain amino acids are the three amino acids (isoleucine, leucine and valine) that are metabolized in the muscles instead of liver, unlike other 17 aminos. The branched-chain aminos can be used to build new protein or be burned as fuel for energy.

Branched-chain amino acids and their powers

Branched-chain amino acids (BCAAs) help decrease exercise-induced muscle damage, increase muscle recovery, and regulate protein synthesis. They may also reduce fatigue. This means being able to train at a higher intensity for a prolonged period of time. BCAAs are most beneficial when included with post-exercise-recovery nutrition, which should begin within 30 minutes of finishing your workout. Consuming protein during this time is critical, and taking advantage of the post-exercise intake provides your muscles with the fuel needed for rebuilding and repair.

BCAAs refer to a group of essential amino acids, including leucine, isoleucine, and valine. Though amino acids are the building blocks of protein, your body can't produce them, so they must be consumed as part of your daily diet. Researchers believe that BCAAs—specifically leucine—are responsible for regulating protein synthesis.

The BCAAs are named like that because they each have a carbon chain which deviates or branches from the main linear carbon backbone. Although structurally similar, with only slight differences in their side chains, they, and their metabolites, have varied functions in protein and neurotransmitter synthesis, and in energy metabolism. BCAAs are important sources of nitrogen for the synthesis of non-dispensable and conditionally dispensable amino acids, such as glutamine and alanine.

These three amino acids are involved in the regulation of protein metabolism, weight loss, body composition. The effects of the BCAAs have recently been the subject of several studies and symposiums. The renewed interest has shed new light on their importance and effects, especially as signaling molecules on protein and energy metabolism.

Earlier studies have shown much of what we need to know about the anabolic and anticatabolic effects of BCAAs, both alone and in concert with other factors such as GH and IGF-1. In heart and skeletal muscle increasing the concentration of the three BCAAs or leucine reproduces the effects of increasing the supply of all amino acids in stimulating protein synthesis and inhibiting protein degradation.

Several studies indicated that leucine is a regulator of protein metabolism by decreasing protein degradation and increasing protein synthesis. It is concluded that leucine decreases protein degradation in humans and that this decrease during leucine infusion contributes to the decrease in plasma essential amino acids. Hormonal response to exercise can be modified by BCAA ingestion and that the anabolic hormones insulin and especially testosterone can be favorably affected when BCAAs is substituted for equivalent amounts of whole-milk proteins. These findings are extremely important and point out the advantages of BCAA supplementation over the use of whole-food proteins and even whole-food protein supplements

Also studies using BCAAs have found them to have a beneficial effect on the synthesis of proteins under special circumstances. The BCAAs (leucine, isoleucine, and valine) are specifically utilized by muscle metabolism, although some evidence indicates their use by other organ tissues.

Leucine and other BCAAs, unlike most other amino acids, are oxidized (used as energy) by muscle cells, and are a source of cellular energy. They are also involved in the glucose alanine cycle. There is a significant activation of BCAA metabolism with prolonged exercise, and current studies indicate that this is more pronounced in endurance-trained subjects than in untrained controls. Plasma concentrations of the BCAAs (leucine, isoleucine, and valine) are more prominently affected than the concentrations of other amino acids by changes in dietary caloric, protein, fat, and carbohydrate intake in humans.

Of the BCAAs, leucine appears to be the most important for athletes. Leucine affects various anabolic hormones and has anabolic and anticatabolic effects. It is also involved in nitrogen metabolism and ammonia removal. A study found that leucine infusion depressed muscle proteolysis. During exercise, protein synthesis decreases as a result of the increased protein degradation and BCAA oxidation. Leucine has been found to stimulate muscle protein synthesis post-exercise. Combined with the aforementioned benefits of all the BCAAs, leucine can help an athlete increase their lean muscle mass. Based on this research, athletes that are trying to cut weight while preserving muscle mass can benefit from supplementation as well those who are trying to increase their lean mass and strength.

Exercise may increase the BCAA requirement. It has been reported that BCAA supplementation before exercise attenuates the breakdown of muscle proteins during exercise in humans and that leucine strongly promotes protein synthesis in skeletal muscle in humans and rats, suggesting that a BCAA supplement may attenuate muscle damage induced by exercise and promote recovery from the damage.

Studies have shown that Branched-chain aminos in are effective for :

Muscle recovery and immune regulation for sports events.

Improving muscle control and mental function in people with advanced liver disease (latent hepatic encephalopathy).

Reducing muscle breakdown during exercise.

Decreasing symptoms associated with mania.

Reducing movements associated with tardive dyskinesia, a disorder associated with the use of antipsychotic medications.

Reducing loss of appetite and improving nutrition in elderly patients on hemodialysis.

There isn't a standardized protocol for BCAA supplementation like there is with protein intake. Many factors affect how much you need. Goals, body mass, age, gender, training experience, and sport are amongst the variables to consider.

Bioavailability of Protein explained – Everything you need to know

Bioavailability means the degree to which your body digests, absorbs and uses food. Dietary protein is not only needed to build bigger muscles, it's also necessary for vibrant-looking skin and lustrous hair. Some protein-rich foods are easier to break down than others, which increases their bioavailability.

Protein bioavailability is the sum total of the three factors:

- The mix of amino acids in the protein -- or in the combination of proteins eaten during the day. Remember, the shortage of an essential amino acid provides a limiting factor on how much of the overall protein can be utilized by the body.

- The structure and size of the protein molecule. The larger and more tightly folded the molecule, the less able the body is to break it down. Large proteins that frequently undergo incomplete digestion include those found in wheat, corn, dairy, and soy.

- The other foods (or components in the protein source itself) that inhibit the breakdown of the protein.

A lot of methods can be used for tracking down bioavailability.

Biological value (BV) measures how much of the protein that you eat gets incorporated into your body tissue. It does so by measuring how much of the nitrogen in the protein you eat is absorbed by the body and then how much is excreted. The assumption is that the difference is what got incorporated into your body protein. This is the most used method of them all.

The Kjeldahl method is the standard for measuring the total protein concentration in food. It provides the number that you normally see on nutrition labels on the side of food packages.

Net protein utilization (NPU) is the ratio of amino acids converted to proteins to the ratio of amino acids supplied in the protein source. Experimentally, this value is calculated by determining the amount of dietary protein you are consuming and then measuring how much nitrogen is excreted. It is significantly affected by the limiting amino acids (as discussed earlier) in the particular food.

Protein Efficiency Ratio (PER) is based on the weight gain of a test subject divided by its intake of a particular food protein during the test period. Theoretically, it is a biological assay of the quality of a particular protein, measured as the gain in weight of an animal per gram of a particular protein eaten. At one time, this was the industry standard, but unfortunately PER is based upon the amino acid requirements of growing rats, which differ noticeably from that of humans.

Protein digestibility corrected amino acid score (PDCAAS) evaluates protein quality based on the amino acid requirements of humans. This is now the preferred standard. Nevertheless, it too has holes. PDCAAS takes no account of where proteins have been digested and cannot account for proteins that are absorbed by bacteria in the digestive tract. PDCAAS is calculated solely on the basis of single protein consumption and therefore once again does not calculate the changes in protein utilization resulting from the intake of complementary protein sources.

Biological Value

As we said, this is the most common used method in calculating protein bioavailability. The BV numbers below demonstrate how easily the body can absorb these protein types.

Meat/dairy/egg vs plant based proteins

Meat/dairy/egg	BV	Plant based proteins	BV
Whey	104	Spirulina	92
Egg	100	Soy	74
Cow's milk	100	Potato	71
Egg white	88	Rice	59
Beef,	80	Wheat	54
Fish	79	Beans	49
Chicken	77	Peanuts	43
Yogurt	42	Pumpkin Seeds	35

Here is also an excellent chart that will help you find out everything you need to know about your plant food in order to properly combine it.

Used shortcuts: *ISO (isoleucine), LEU (leucine), LYS(lysine), MET (methionine), PHE (phenylalanine), TRP (tryptophan), VAL (valine), HIS (histidine), THR (threonine)*

Basic Whole Foods Commonly Found in Vegetarian or Vegan	Limiting Amino Acids	High Amino Acids	Servi Size	Calorie Per Serving	Gr Per Servi	Gr Protein Per 100 g 100g	Protein as % of Calorie	Combine With
Legumes: Beans and Lentils,								
Lentils	MET-TRP	ISO-LYS	1 Cup	115	17.13	8.97	24.3	grains
Mung Bean	TRP	ISO-LYS	1 Cup	105	13.57	7.54	24.3	nuts
Chick Pea	MET-TRP	ISO-LYS	1 Cup	180	15.65	9.54	19.4	seeds
Black Eyed Pea	ISO	ISO-LYS	1 Cup	115	12.98	7.68	23.7	veggies
Black Bean	MET-LEU	ISO-LYS	1 Cup	115	12.49	7.26		
Fava Bean		THR	1 Cup	109	12.85	7.56	23.7	
Kidney Bean		ISO-LYS	1 Cup	126	14.83	8.62		
Lima Bean	TRP	PHE	1 Cup	113	10 g	7.75	20	
Miso			1	199	2 g	11.69		
Pigeon Peas			1 Cup	170	9.12	5.96		
Pinto Beans	MET-TRP	ISO-LYS	1 Cup		15			
Soybean	MET	TRP- LEU	1 Cup	172	29.77	16.54	39.4	
Soymilk	VAL	TRP - LEU	1 Cup	45	6.62	2.7	30	
Split Peas	MET-TRP		1 Cup					
Tempeh	VAL		3 oz		15 g	17	36	
Tofu	MET	HIS	1/2	151	20		61.2	
TVP	MET		1/2		16			
Seeds, Raw								Combine
Flax Seeds (whole)	LYS-ISO	THR	1	44	1.5 g	18.29	12.5	With
Hemp Seeds	VAL	MET	1			29.9		grains,
Pumpkin Seeds	LYS-ISO	MET	1	46	2 g	24.54		legumes
Sesame Seeds	LYS	VAL- HIS	1		1.6 g	17.73	7.9	veggies
Sunflower Seeds	LYS	VAL- HIS	1	46	1.8 g	20.78	19.8	fruit
Tahini (sesame seed	LYS	VAL- HIS	1	47		17		
Nuts, Raw								Combine
Almond	ISO-VAL	MET	1/2		3 g	16.8	9.6	With
Brazil Nut	ISO-LYS	MET				14.8	7.9	grains,
Cashews			1 Oz.		2.5 g	17.4	11.1	legumes
Coconut	LYS					6.6	3.9	veggies
Hazelnut	THR-ISO	PHE				19.9	11.7	fruit
Peanut Butter	LYS-TRP	PHE	1		4 g			
Peanuts	LYS-TRP	PHE	1 oz.		7 g			
Pecan	VAL					6.25	7.8	
Pistachio	LYS-THR	PHE				18.9	11	
Walnut	ISO-LYS		1/2 oz (7			15.6	8.2	

Grains, Cooked Unless Otherwise								
Amaranth								Combine
Barley - Hulled	ISO LYS	MET	1 cup		3.64	2.25	11.8	With
Barley - Pearled			1 cup	193	3.55	2.26		legumes
Bulgar	LYS		1 cup	151	5.61	3.06	11.4	nuts
Brown Rice	VAL	MET	1 cup	216	5.03	2.56	7.2	seeds
Buckwheat Groats	ISO LYS		1 cup	155	5.68	3.37		veggies
Cornmeal whole	LYS TRP	MET	1 cup	*180	4.42	1.84	7.3	fruit
Couscous cooked			1 cup	176	5.95	3.79		
Farina	LYS ISO		1 cup		3.11	1.24		
Japanese Soba Noodles	TRP MET		1 cup	113	5.77	3.06		
Kamut cooked	LYS TRP		1 cup	251	11.25	6.1		
Millet cooked	LYS ISO		1 cup	207	6.09	3.5	10.2	
Oat Bran		MET						
Oats cooked	ISO LYS		1 cup	*200	4.98	2.13	12	
Quick Rice (Parboiled)	ISO LYS		1 cup	194	4.6	2.66	7.6	
Quinoa cooked	PHE THR	MET-TRP	1 cup	222	8.14	4.4	12.6	
Pasta-Wheat, cooked,			1 cup	221	8.12			
Rice Noodles cooked		MET		192	1.6			
Seitan (Wheat Gluten)	ISO		3 oz	120	22	75.58		
Teff cooked	LYS TRP		1 cup	249	9.76			
Triticale Flour (wh gr)			1 cup	439	17.3			
Wheat Bran (dry)		MET	1 cup	125	9.02	15.55	13.6	
Wheat Germ (dry)	LYS TRP	MET-TRP	1 cup	414	26.62	23.15		
Wheat Rolled cooked	LYS	MET	1 cup		3.7	1.53		
Wheat sprouted	LYS		1 cup	214	8.09			
White Flour (wheat)	LYS THR	MET	1 cup	*480	12.91	9.71		
White Rice cooked	ISO LYS	MET	1 cup	194	4.2	2.66	7.1	
Whole Wheat Bread	LYS		1 slice		4 g			
Whole Wheat Flour	LYS ISO		1 cup	407	16.44	13.7	13.1	
Wild Rice cooked		MET-TRP	1 cup	166	6.54	3.99		

Vegetables With A High Protein								Combine
Asparagus	LYS		1/2 Cup	10	2.16	2.1	30.1	With
Avocado			1					nuts
Beet Greens			1/2 Cup	20	3.7	2.57		seeds
Broccoli	MET	ISO-LYS	1/2 Cup	25	3.2	4.29	28.4	grain
Chard				17	1.15	1.88		legumes
Collard Greens				25	1.9	2.11		
Corn on the cob			1 ear	48	1.5	3.5		
Corn Kernels Frozen			1/2 Cup	60	2.05	3.02		
Edamame (green	MET		1/2 Cup	65	6	10.25		
Green Peas	MET-TRP	LEU-LYS	1/2 Cup	61	3.91	4.47		
Hubbard Squash			1/2 Cup	51	2.5	2.4		
Kale	MET-TRP		1/2 Cup	18	1.25	1.9		
Mung Bean Sprouts	MET-TRP		1/2 Cup	11.5	1.26	2		
Mushroom (cloud -	ISO		1/2 Cup	40	1.3	9.25		
Mushroom (Crimini -	MET-TRP	LEU-LYS	1/2 Cup	12	1.09	2.5		
Mushroom (oyster -	MET-TRP		1/2 cup	33	2.45	3.31		
Mushrooms (Portobella	MET-TRP		1/2 Cup	21	2.53	4.27		
Mustard Greens	MET-TRP		1/2 Cup	10.5	1.58	2.26		
Potato Flour (dry)	LYS-TRP		1 Cup	571	11.04	6.9		
Potato peeled	LYS-TRP		1			1.3	4.2	
Potato w/skin baked	LYS-TRP		1	161	4.32	2.5	6.9	
Salsify			1/2 Cup	46	1.6	2.73		
Spinach	MET-ISO	LEU-LYS	1/2 Cup	21	2.62	2.97	25.66	
Spirolina (dried)	MET	LEU-ISO	1 Tblsp	20	4.02	3.5		
Sugar Snap Peas			1/2 Cup	33.5	2.61	3.27		
Fruit:								Combine
Dates (dried)	ISO					2.7	3.1	With
Figs (dried)	ISO					1.2	6.1	legumes
Bananas		TRP						nuts, seeds
								veggies

The plants will do more than fine - High protein plant based sources

If there is a chance that you want to base you diet on plant sourced food, but you are not sure which one is the best for you, we give you a list of plant food that has a high BV among other values.

Spirulina

Spirulina is a type of blue-green algae that's very dense in protein and an excellent source of some vitamins and minerals. Spirulina is composed of about 70 percent complete protein in its natural state, which is higher than any other unprocessed food. The biological value of spirulina is about 92, in part because it doesn't have cellulose in its cell walls, which allows your body to easily break it down. The main issues with spirulina are that it is relatively expensive, not very tasty and can accumulate toxins from polluted water.

Soy

Soy is the most widely used vegetable protein source. The soybean, from the legume family, was first chronicled in China in the year 2838 B.C. and was considered to be as valuable as wheat, barley, and rice as a nutritional staple

Soy's quality makes it a very attractive alternative for those seeking non-animal sources of

protein in their diet and those who are lactose intolerant. Soy is a complete protein with a high

concentration of BCAA's. There have been many reported benefits related to soy proteins relating to health and performance (including reducing plasma lipid profiles, increasing LDL-cholesterol oxidation and reducing blood pressure).

The soybean can be separated into three distinct categories; flour, concentrates, and isolates. Soy flour can be further divided into natural or full-fat (contains natural oils), defatted (oils removed), and lecithinated (lecithin added) forms . Of the three different categories of soy protein products, soy flour is the least refined form. It is commonly found in baked goods. Another product of soy flour is called textured soy flour. This is primarily used for processing as a meat extender.

Soy concentrate was developed in the late 1960s and early 1970s and is made from defatted soybeans. While retaining most of the bean's protein content, concentrates do not contain as much soluble carbohydrates as flour, making it more palatable. Soy concentrate has a high digestibility and is found in nutrition bars, cereals, and yogurts. Isolates are the most refined soy protein product containing the greatest concentration of protein, but unlike flour and concentrates, contain no dietary fiber. They are very digestible and easily introduced into foods such as sports drinks and health beverages as well as infant formulas.

For centuries, soy has been part of a human diet. Epidemiologists were most likely the first to recognize soy's benefits to overall health when considering populations with a high intake of soy. These populations shared lower incidences in certain cancers, decreased cardiac conditions, and improvements in menopausal symptoms and osteoporosis in women.

Also there is a lot of debate in comparing whey and soy proteins. So we will try to do shed some light on that as well. Although there are some benefits in whey protein, he has a lot of more side effects and bad qualities attached to him than soy protein. Because whey protein is pasteurized, some of the growth factors and proteins found in it may be damaged, making them useless for our bodies. Whey protein can contain estrogenic chemicals that the cattle industry uses to help with weight gain. People who are lactose intolerant may have issues consuming whey protein so it can lead to intestinal issues such as bloating and gas.

Hemp Seed Protein

Hemp seed protein has some unique features. First, 65% of the total protein content of hemp seed comes from the globular protein edestin, which is easily digested, absorbed, and utilized by the human body. As a side note, it closely resembles the globulin found in human blood plasma, which is vital to maintaining a healthy immune system. As such, edestin has the unique ability to stimulate the manufacture of antibodies against foreign invaders. It is also hypoallergenic.

Grains and beans

Number of grains and beans are complete proteins and can serve as a foundational protein for vegetarian diets. But they tend to be unbalanced in their amino acid ratios. This means that you have to eat them in proper combinations.

Rice and Pea

Rice protein is high in cysteine and methionine, but tends to be low in lysine. Yellow pea protein, tends to be low in the sulfur containing amino acids, cysteine and methionine, but high in lysine. And when used in combination, rice protein and yellow pea protein offer a protein efficiency ratio that begins to rival dairy and egg -- but without their potential to promote allergic reactions. In addition, the texture of pea protein helps smooth out the "chalkiness" of rice protein. Like rice protein, it is hypoallergenic and easily digested. On a different note, the rice/pea combo also has a nice branch chain amino acid profile -- only slightly less than whey.

Amaranth seed

Ancient amaranth grains still used to this day include the three species, Amaranthus caudatus, Amaranthus cruentus, and Amaranthus hypochondriacus. Although amaranth was cultivated on a large scale in ancient Mexico, Guatemala, and Peru, nowadays it is only cultivated on a small scale there, along with India, China, Nepal, and other tropical countries; thus, there is potential for further cultivation in those countries, as well as in the U.S. In a 1977 article in Science, amaranth was described as "the crop of the future. There are some great positive things about it : It is easily harvested.

Its seeds are a good source of protein. Compared to grains, amaranth is unusually rich in the essential amino acid lysine. Common grains such as wheat and corn are comparatively rich in amino acids that amaranth lacks; thus, amaranth and grains can complement each other.

The seeds of Amaranthus species contain about thirty percent more protein than cereals like rice, sorghum and rye. In cooked and edible forms, amaranth is competitive with wheat germ and oats - higher in some nutrients, lower in others.

It is easy to cook.

As befits its weedy life history, amaranth grains grow very rapidly and their large seedheads can weigh up to 1 kilogram and contain a half-million seeds in three species of amaranth.

Quinoa

Quinoa grain has been called a superfood, a term which is not in common use by dietitians and nutrition scientists. Protein content is very high for a cereal/pseudo-cereal (14% by mass), but not as high as most beans and legumes. This includes a "low gluten content that appears to be well tolerated when consumed at normal levels by people with celiac disease. The protein content per 100 calories is higher than brown rice, potatoes, barley and millet, but is less than wild rice and oats. Nutritional evaluations indicate that quinoa is a source of complete protein. Other sources claim its protein is not complete but relatively high in essential amino acids

Quinoa is a rich source of the B vitamins thiamine, riboflavin, vitamin B6, and folate and is a rich source of the dietary minerals iron, magnesium, phosphorus, and zinc. Quinoa is also a good source of the B vitamins niacin and pantothenic acid, vitamin E, and the dietary mineral potassium. The pseudo cereal contains a modest amount of calcium, and thus is useful for vegans and those who are lactose intolerant. It is gluten-free and considered easy to digest.

Lentils

The lentil (Lens culinaris) is an edible pulse. It is a bushy annual plant of the legume family, known for its lens-shaped seeds. It is about 40 cm (16 in) tall, and the seeds grow in pods, usually with two seeds in each. With 26% of total food content from protein, lentils have the third-highest level of protein, by weight, of any legume or nut, after soybeans and hemp Red (or pink) lentils contain a lower concentration of fiber than green lentils (11% versus 31%).

The low levels of readily digestible starch (5%), and high levels of slowly digested starch (30%), make lentils of potential value to people with diabetes.

Pea protein powder

Pea protein powder provides a delicious alternative source of protein for anyone but especially for vegetarians, vegans or those following restricted diets. It is entirely gluten-free, soy-free and dairy-free. It provides an array of benefits for health and fitness.

Yellow peas supply a unique array of essential and non essential amino acids, the building blocks of bodily tissue and muscles. Being especially high in lysine and arginine, pea protein is especially beneficial for active lifestyles.As we said before Lysine cannot be made in the body and must therefore be consumed through the diet.

 Plant-based foods provide a source of non-heme iron for the body to absorb. Pea protein provides 30% of the iron required per day in a single serving. Combining this product with citric acids (e.g. lemon/lime/orange juice) will optimize the absorption of the iron content. In unrestricted diets, iron absorption can also be enhanced when consumed with animal-based protein. Iron absorption can be inhibited when consumed with coffee, tea or foods rich in calcium.

Pea protein powder provides a supplemental source of dietary protein for vegetarians and/or vegans who cannot use animal proteins. Due to advances in protein extraction methods, yellow pea protein can successfully be extracted from the legume. Since protein is an essential macro-nutrient often lacking in vegetarians, protein powders can help fill the nutritional gap.

Some individuals simply cannot tolerate egg, milk and soy-derived protein due to allergies. For example, the milk sugar called lactose can cause severe allergic reactions that result in unwanted gastrointestinal side effects like nausea, bloating, diarrhea or vomiting. Yellow pea protein powder is suitable for almost any user. It also contains no gluten, the wheat protein that some manufacturers add to powders or products. Most yellow proteins are organic and contain little or no artificial colors, sweeteners or fillers.

Brown Rice protein powder

Brown rice protein isn't a complete protein by itself, meaning you need to buy a powder that contains enhanced amino acids—or you need to pair it with something, like tofu, quinoa or beans, that will round out the nutrients you need. Still, it has its own unique benefits. It's high in fiber, gluten-free, lactose-free and full of B vitamins, which help out with muscle metabolism and growth. Brown rice protein is labeled as hypoallergenic, so it's less likely to irritate your system or cause an allergic reaction.

Combining plant based protein sources to reach peak bioavailability

Protein combining (also protein complementing) is a dietary strategy for protein nutrition by using complementary sources to optimize biological value. If you want to boost your protein level, only one type of meal isn't enough for that. You need to have balanced diet so your protein level is on the top. Lot of people are worried that they may lack some of essential amino acids if they are vegans. But that isn't true, this is one of the oldest myths related to vegetarianism and was disproved long ago.. Eating a variety of plants can serve as a well-balanced and complete source of amino acids. It is very easy for a vegan diet to meet the recommendations for protein. Nearly all vegetables, beans, grains, nuts, and seeds contain some much protein. Fruits, sugars, fats, and alcohol do not provide much protein, so a diet based only on these foods would have a good chance of being too low in protein. However, not many vegans we know live on only bananas, hard candy, margarine, and beer. Vegans eating varied diets containing vegetables, beans, grains, nuts, and seeds rarely have any difficulty getting enough protein as long as their diet contains enough energy (calories) to maintain weight.

Do not confuse combining foods to get complete proteins for the dietary trend called "food combining." The two differ in both theory and practice. The dietary trend of food combining requires that all food intake be scrutinized and that specific combinations be eaten in a certain order and even at a certain time of day. This type of eating is supposed to result in digestive benefits, including easier digestion, more complete absorption of nutrients and easier breakdown of fats and carbohydrates.

On the other hand, combining foods for complete meatless proteins is a process with the goal of supplying balanced nutrition for meals that do not contain meat. There is no digestive or nutritive goal beyond making complete proteins from vegetable, grain, bean or legume, and seed or nut combinations. Though these foods are healthy, by themselves they cannot supply complete proteins.

There has long been speculation as to whether or not it is necessary to combine proteins within a single meal to complete them. Some say it is, but a position paper on vegetarian diets by the American Dietetic Association states that plant protein can meet dietary protein requirements when a variety of plant foods is consumed and a person's diet has sufficient calories. In addition, research indicates that plant foods eaten throughout the day can provide the diet with all essential amino acids. Further, the proteins do not have to be eaten together in a single meal.

List One	List Two	List Three
(foods low in sulfur)	(foods low in tryptophan)	(foods low in lysine)
Green beans	Barley	Almonds
Asparagus	Mushrooms	Pumpkin seeds
Broccoli	Chard	Pecans
Potatoes	Green peas	Yams
Lentils	Garbanzo beans	Brown rice
Soybeans	Brown rice	Corn

Combining Whole Grains With Legumes

Legumes provide an essential amino acid called lysine, which is low in many grains. Whole grains provide methionine and cysteine, which are low in legumes, or beans, peas, lentils and peanuts. You can combine grains and legumes to make high-quality proteins. Examples include black bean and corn salad with brown rice, pinto beans in a whole-wheat pita, split-pea soup with barley and peanut butter on whole-wheat toast. Whole grains are higher in protein than refined grains, such as white bread and pasta.

Combining Nuts and Seeds With Legumes or Grains

Combining legumes with sunflower seeds, sesame seeds or nuts, such as pecans, walnuts, almonds and pistachios, provides complete proteins. For a snack, you could have trail mix with nuts, peanuts and sunflower seeds or vegetables and hummus dip, which has garbanzo beans and tahini, or sesame seed paste. You can also combine grains with nuts or seeds. Examples include oatmeal with sliced almonds or other nuts, and whole-grain bread with nuts and seeds.

As we said before, it is not necessary to have complete proteins at every meal. As long as you are accumulating a variety of proteins from the sources in the list below daily, your body can make the proteins it needs for good health. The body pulls amino acids from it's amino acid pool to make any type of protein the body needs. The pool is made from digested proteins that come from your diet and those that the body makes. This list will show you how to create complete proteins at any meal. Combining the right plant foods together in one meal will help form a complete protein source .There are different combination's of plant foods that can be selected so you can choose which food you prefer to eat

The next charts will give you some more specific instructions how to reach peak bioavailability.

GROUP #1

"Breads, Cereals, Grains"

Whole Grain Breads such as rye, wheat, oat, rice, spelt, quinoa, Long Grain Brown Rice, Whole wheat products & Whole grain cereals

these include: breakfast cereal, pasta, spaghetti, noodles, wheat products, flour products, etc.

Any item from **group # 1** above to be combined with any item from one of the three groups below.

Group # 2	Group # 3	Group # 4
"Legumes" Peas, Beans & Lentils:	**"Vegetables"** Leafy Green and Cruciferous Vegetables	**Nuts & Seed** Almonds, Pumpkin Seeds, Walnuts, Cashews
including all dried beans & peas - black, kidney, pinto, black eyed peas, runner,chick peas, sweet green peas, processed peas, baked beans, beansprouts	including frozen vegetables	Peanuts, etc Sunflower, Sesame & other seeds

The top five plant based food combinations

One more great thing we would like to share with you are food combinations that make up a full amino spectrum and are great protein sources. Every single one of these combinations contains all essential amino acids, and makes a complete protein.

Peanuts & Whole Wheat

According to Diane Birt, P.D., a professor at Iowa State University and a food synergy expert, the specific amino acids absent in wheat are actually present in peanuts. You need, and very rarely receive in one meal, the complete chain of amino acids (the best form of protein) to build and maintain muscle, especially as you get older. In short, while this combo exhibits only what Birt calls a "loose definition" of food synergy, it gives good evidence that a peanut-butter sandwich isn't junk food if it's prepared with whole-wheat bread (not white) and eaten in moderation (once a day).

So enjoy a peanut-butter sandwich right after a workout instead of drinking a terrible gym-rat shake. Just make sure the peanut butter doesn't have added sugar, chemical ingredients you can't pronounce, or cartoon characters on the label.

Rice and Beans

This combination is very nutritious. Rice is rich in starch, an excellent source of energy. Rice also has iron, vitamin B and protein. Beans also contain a good amount of iron and an even greater amount of protein than rice. Also the beans are full of fiber, potassium, folate, iron, manganese and magnesium, and they are cholesterol and fat-free. They are a super food.

Together they make up a complete protein, which provides each of the amino acids the body cannot make for itself. In addition, rice and beans are common and affordable ingredients, often available in difficult economic times.

This is a winning combination, just as long as the ratio to beans and rice is not too off balance.

Hummus and Wheat

Hummus is loaded with protein, courtesy of its two main ingredients, chickpeas and tahini. The protein in wheat is similar to that of rice, in that it's only deficient in lysine. But chickpeas have plenty of lysine. So that's a perfect reason to combine hummus with various wheat meals.

Chickpeas have a similar amino acid profile to most legumes, so don't be afraid to experiment with hummus made from cannellini, edamame, or other kinds of beans.

Spirulina with Grains or Nuts

Spirulina contains the most powerful combination of nutrients ever known in any grain, herb or food. It's an exceptionally good protein source, and contains most of the essential minerals and vitamins, particularly iron and the B vitamins, Spirulina beta carotene is ten times more concentrated than carrots.

But contrary to popular belief, this member of the algae family is not a complete protein, since it's lacking in methionine and cysteine. Adding something with plenty of these amino acids, such as grains, oats, nuts, or seeds, and you have yourself a complete protein.

Corn and Beans

Beans are more popular in the combination with rice, but you don't have to go with the popular always. There are more combinations than just one. Neither beans nor corn alone, of course, is such a complete food because neither is a complete protein. But paired, these two make a complete protein.

Beans contain all the essential amino acids but one, methionine, which just happens to be the amino acid that corn *does* have plenty. Corn also contains a lot of B vitamins, dietary fiber and the essential minerals, magnesium and phosphorus. Together, a mixture of two parts corn and one part beans is almost equal in protein quality to fresh milk.

Now we come to the delicious part - High protein meals

We have all been there. You want to cook, but you have no clue what to prepare. Fear no more. We will share some recipes with you for high protein meals. And the best of all, you don't need any animal products to make them. Trust me, they are even more delicious.

Seitan Roast Stuffed with Walnuts, Dried Cranberries, and Mushrooms

Protein amount: 39,1g

Ingredients:

Stuffing

1/2 large onion, chopped

1 rib celery, chopped

4 ounces mushrooms, sliced or chopped

1 teaspoon dried thyme

1/2 teaspoon rubbed sage

generous grinding of pepper

3 ounces whole wheat bread (about 2 slices), cut into small cubes

1/3 cup dried cranberries or cherries

1/4 cup chopped walnuts

1 teaspoon whole chia seeds or ground flax seed

1 tablespoon soy sauce

1/2 cup water (more as needed)

Seitan

2 cups vital wheat gluten (10 ounces)

1/4 cup nutritional yeast

1 teaspoon dried thyme

1 teaspoon rubbed sage

1 teaspoon marjoram

1/3 cup quinoa flakes or quick oatmeal

1 teaspoon chia seed or ground flaxseeds

1 1/2 cup vegetable broth

1 cup great northern beans, cooked

2 tablespoons soy sauce

1 clove garlic, peeled

1 tablespoon tahini (preferred) or other nut butter

Baking Broth

1/2 cup vegetable broth

1 tablespoon soy sauce

1/2 teaspoon dark sesame oil (optional)

Instructions

Stuffing:

Sauté the onion and celery in a non-stick skillet until onion is becoming translucent. Add the mushrooms, thyme, sage, and a generous grating of black pepper and cover. Cook until mushrooms exude their juices, about 3 minutes. Add the remaining ingredients along with enough water to moisten the stuffing but not make it soaking wet. Remove from heat and keep covered.

Seitan:

In a mixing bowl, combine the dry ingredients (vital wheat gluten through chia seeds). Place the 1 1/2 cups of broth, white beans, soy sauce, and garlic in blender and process until liquefied. Make a well in the center of the dry ingredients, add the bean mixture, and stir until gluten is completely moistened. Drizzle the tahini over the top and knead it into the dough. Keep kneading until dough holds together in a ball. Set aside while you make the broth.

Broth:

Heat all ingredients until hot but not boiling.

Preparation

Preheat oven to 400. Lightly oil an oval or rectangular baking dish, 11-13 inches long and 6-8 inches wide. (Your seitan will expand to fit it, so try not to use a very wide dish.) Line your work surface with plastic wrap, parchment paper, or waxed paper. Place the dough in the center, cover it with plastic wrap, and roll out the seitan, making sure that it is the same thickness in all places, until it's about 9×13 (an inch or so either way doesn't matter, but make sure it's not longer than your pan). Spread the stuffing evenly, leaving a 1-inch margin on all sides. Lift up the plastic wrap on one of the long edges and roll the seitan up like a jelly roll. (Alternatively, arrange the stuffing in a horizontal line across the middle of the seitan and bring one long edge up and over it to the other side.) Pinch the ends sealed first and then pinch well to seal the long seam. Take care to make sure that the edges are completely sealed and no gaps or stuffing shows. Lift the seitan roll carefully and place seam-side down in the prepared casserole dish. Pour the baking broth over it, add rosemary, and cover tightly. If the dish doesn't have a cover, use aluminum foil to cover tightly. (Did I mention "tightly?" Tightly! I enclosed even the bottom of the dish in foil.)

Bake for 25 minutes. Remove from oven, baste with broth, recover tightly, and bake for another 25 minutes. Baste again and return to oven uncovered for about 30 minutes. Baste 2 or 3 times as it's cooking. Seitan is done when top seems firm and brown and the broth has evaporated. You can test it by cutting a small slit in the middle; if it is doughy rather than firm, return to the oven.

Remove from the oven and let cool for 5-10 minutes. Transfer carefully to a cutting board or serving platter and cut into 1/2-inch slices.

Bean Burritos

Ingredients:

1 tablespoon canola oil

1 garlic clove, minced

1/2 teaspoon chipotle chile powder*

1/4 teaspoon salt

1/3 cup water

1 (15-ounce) can organic black beans, drained

1 (15-ounce) can organic kidney beans, drained

3 tablespoons salsa

6 (10-inch) flour tortillas

1 cup (4 ounces) preshredded 4-cheese Mexican blend cheese

1 1/2 cups chopped plum tomato (about 3)

1 1/2 cups shredded romaine lettuce

6 tablespoons thinly sliced green onions (optional)

6 tablespoons light sour cream (optional)

Preparation:

Heat oil in a large nonstick skillet over medium heat. Add garlic to pan; cook 1 minute, stirring frequently. Stir in chile powder and salt; cook 30 seconds, stirring constantly. Stir in 1/3 cup water and beans; bring to a boil. Reduce heat, and simmer 10 minutes. Remove from heat; stir in salsa. Partially mash bean mixture with a fork.

Layer a dinner plate with a damp paper towel. Place a tortilla on the paper towel. Cover with another damp paper towel. Continue layering tortillas with paper towels until you have as many as desired. Warm tortillas according to package directions, about 30 seconds in the microwave. Spoon about 1/3 cup bean mixture into center of each tortilla. Top each serving with about 2 1/2 tablespoons cheese, 1/4 cup tomato, 1/4 cup lettuce, 1 tablespoon onions, and 1 tablespoon sour cream; roll up.

Vegetarian pepperoni burrito

Protein amount: 35g

Ingredients:

several slices of vegetarian pepperoni

1/4 cup soy mozzarella cheese

1/4 cup spaghetti sauce, heated

1 flour tortilla

Preparation:

Lay out several slices of veggie pepperoni on a flour tortilla, spoon spaghetti sauce on top and sprinkle cheese over all. Roll into a burrito. Simple, right?

Burgers

Protein amount: 36g

Ingredients:

2 cups TVP

6 tablespoons taco seasoning

2 cups vegetable broth

1/2 cup oil

4 cups cooked pinto beans (2 15-oz cans)

2 bunches fresh cilantro leaves

4 cups vital wheat gluten

1 1/2 cups nondairy sour cream

Instructions:

Heat vegie broth to boiling point and in a very large bowl, pour over the TVP. Cover and let stand 10 minutes.

In food processor, using the small bowl, whirl the oil and cilantro, adding the leaves in small batches. Add this, along with taco seasoning and beans to the presoaked TVP and stir in.

Add the wheat gluten one cup at a time, mixing with your hands. Once thoroughly mixed, add the sour cream and mix again using your hand.

Set oven for 350 degrees.

Shape dough into 12 burgers and set on oiled cookie sheets. Bake 20 minutes, then turn burgers (at this stage be careful not to break them) and bake 15 minutes more.

www.ingramcontent.com/pod-product-compliance
Lightning Source LLC
Chambersburg PA
CBHW070845290526

45795CB00002B/993